WHAT READERS ARE SAYING ABOUT INTERMITTENT FASTING

Such an informative book! This book packs so much info and makes it super clear and concise. If you want to give intermittent fasting a try this is the book for you!

— Cody, Amazon Verified Purchase Review

This book offers a complete and comprehensive study about intermittent fasting and provides helpful information to unleashing your body's full potential. It will help you burn fat and build lean muscle. I will recommend this book to everyone.

— Arturo, Amazon Verified Purchase Review

While reading the first chapter of the book I knew it was a gem! What will separate this book from other intermittent guides is how it first tries to establish the correct mindset of the reader. It helps the reader understand goal setting and how the most important part is psychology before the mechanics. It does a great job of explaining what intermittent fasting is, how to build muscle while intermittent fasting, and also supplies an exercise plan! Please do yourself a favor and buy this book.

— Mackenzie, Amazon Verified Purchase Review

A well explained and complete guide to intermittent fasting! I am new to intermittent fasting and this book has been my guide. I'm glad I bought this book by Noah Lively! 5 stars!

— Jasmine, Amazon Verified Purchase Review

INTERMITTENT FASTING

OTHER BOOKS BY NOAH LIVELY

Meal Prep: The Ultimate Guide to Create Your Own Recipies, Lose Weight, Build Muscle, & Live Healthy

Intermittent Fasting

Fasting

Ultimate Guide to Lose Fat, Build Muscle, & Feel Your Best

NOAH LIVELY

I dedicate this book to all of those not willing to settle. It is you that will change the world.

YOUR FREE DOWNLOADS

WANT **FREE** RESOURCES TO HELP YOU
REACH YOUR GOALS **FASTER**?

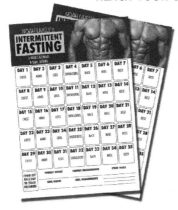

1. TRAINING CALENDAR

DOWNLOAD & PRINT
THE FREE GOAL SETTING &
ACCOUNTABILITY CALENDAR!

2. PRINTED TRAINING PROGRAM

TAKE THE PROGRAM WITH YOU.
INCLUDES VOLUME TRACKER. HELPS YOU:
+ REMEMBER YOUR LIFTS
+ GET STRONGER
+ BUILD MUSCLE

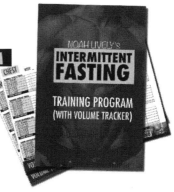

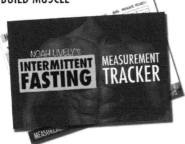

3. MEASUREMENT TRACKER

+ MAKE PROGRESS EVERY WEEK
+ SEE YOUR RESULTS OVER TIME

DOWNLOAD LINK: WWW.BIT.LY/2LWKI92

CONTENTS

INTRODUCTION

"To lengthen thy Life, lessen thy meals." **~ Benjamin Franklin**

Have you ever struggled to lose weight? Do you feel like it's hard to add muscle? Have you ever struggled to find your motivation? Do you feel overwhelmed and don't know where to start?

If you answered yes to any of those questions, I wrote this book for you.

We live in a world filled with more information than ever. Yet, people are more confused than ever. I have seen so many people try to master their weight and nutrition. But time and time again, they fail. No matter how hard they try, the weight comes crawling back and motivation is lost. Then they quit.

After a few months, they decide to try again only to experience the same cycle. This happens time and time again until they are convinced that complacency is their destiny, but it doesn't have to be.

How do I know this? I've been there before.

I was 30 pounds overweight and tried everything to lose it. I read every article I could get my hands on and that confused me more than ever. First, I thought I had a slow metabolism (I'll talk more about that in the **myth's section**). Then, I thought I had problems digesting specific foods. I cut fats out of my diet - only to get a blood test that suggested I add it back. I cut out carbs only to lose muscle, strength, and endurance.

I was frustrated to say the least. Maybe you can relate.

That is when I came across intermittent fasting. I was desperate. I had tried everything else so I decided to give this one last shot. What else did I have to lose?

The results were nothing short of amazing. I lost 30 pounds in just 5 months.

Now, I know many of you may think I'm lying and it's another one of those false claims that try to manipulate you to buy a product. However, I have no reason to lie to you. If you're reading this, you have already purchased this product and are (hopefully) committed to seeing yourself change.

Weight loss is simpler than you think (I'll explain this in detail in **Chapter 5**).

Once I lost 30 pounds and discovered the right strategies to lose weight, I wanted to see if it worked for other people. So I got some people to follow the same strategies outlines in this book. They did. Everyone who implemented what I'm going to tell you lost weight - and it was the easiest thing for them to do.

Get ready to be set free from the bondage that food may have.
Get ready to take control of your weight and your life.

In this book, I'm going to show you how to lose stubborn fat. I'll reveal critical keys to motivation; give you tips that make fasting easy; help you build strong, hard muscle; and challenge you to start right away.

So let's get started. Flip this page and let's start our journey together.

- Noah Lively

CHAPTER 1: HOW TO STAY MOTIVATED

The Choice Everyone Must Make

People often start a new fitness plan or diet only to fail a few weeks later. This can happen for a number of reasons. I hear it all the time:

- I don't have the time.
- This is too hard.
- I've tried everything
- If only I had their genetics.

The list goes on and on. My goal, however, is to ensure this doesn't happen to you.

I want to challenge you today. I want to challenge you to make a decision that you will commit to the process. Choose now – will you give yourself this gift? You will be amazed at the results you can achieve if you just commit.

Motivation is critical to the weight loss win. To ensure you follow through, you must achieve clarity. Clarity is power. We can achieve this clarity by answering a few questions. Take some time and ask yourself the following:

1: Why do you want this?
  o *Examples may include: I want to impress my husband. I want to look my best. I want to fit into my clothes. I want to make my girlfriend proud. I want to feel more confident. I want to prove that I have control.*

2: Why is this a MUST for you?
  o When something becomes a *must*, it will get done. No exceptions.

You *must* work. You *must* sleep at night. Take some time and write down some reasons why this is a *must* for you.

3: What will happen if you do NOT do this?
- o Most of us are motivated by pain. It's why we procrastinate. We don't like doing a big project because of the pain associated with working on that project. However, we would find time to complete the project if it's due the next day. Why? Because the pain of not completing the project just became more than the pain of doing it. This is a powerful concept.

- o Write down some reasons why it would bring pain if you do *not* commit to this.

Your answers to these questions will give you the emotional juice needed to push through when you don't feel like it. If you haven't done so already, grab a piece of paper and write your answers down. Don't continue until you have.

Did you do it?
Take that note and stick it to your bathroom mirror. Every morning when you wake up, read them. Say them aloud. Remind yourself why you are doing this. Believe that you can do this.

Long-Term vs. Short-Term Thinking
People tend to give up when something doesn't go the way they planned. I want you to remember this is a marathon, not a sprint.

People often approach me with these crazy weight loss goals. When I hear them, I already know there is no way they will achieve them. Before they have even started, they have set themselves up for failure.

No matter who you are, there is no way you can lose 30 pounds in a week. Even if you ate nothing and ran all day long, you wouldn't even come close. Not to mention that this strategy is not sustainable and would be harmful to your health.

When it comes to losing weight, the most important element is to have a healthy perspective. Understand that you may not lose all your weight in a week, you may not build all the muscle you want in a week, but you *will be* one week closer to your ultimate goal.

4

The key in all of this is to focus on the process, not the result. Why? Because it is the process you choose that determines the result you get.

When most people set goals, they set result-orientated goals. Examples of result-orientated goals would include, "I want to lose 10 pounds", or "I want to pick up 5 pounds of lean muscle." While all these goals are great, understand that result-orientated goals need process-orientated habits if you ever plan on achieving them.

Instead of saying, "I want to lose 10 pounds in 5 weeks," set a process-orientated goal by saying, "I choose to follow my meal plan every day this week," or "I choose to work out 5 times this week."

If you complete the process, you are succeeding – even if you don't achieve the result.

The Ultimate Way to Overcome Excuses

*"Whether you believe you can or can't, you're right." - **Henry Ford***

Our failures are most often a result of our limiting beliefs. This is something I am guilty of all the time. I often allow myself to believe the lies I tell myself. I tell myself, "I don't have the time. I'll never look the way I want. I will always be this way."

The challenge is our actions follow our beliefs. What you choose to believe is what you'll become. The lies you believe will be come a self-fulfilling prophecy.

The best technique is to take those lies, those disempowering statements you believe, and turn them into empowering ones. Instead of saying, "I don't have the time," ask, "What can I do with the time that I do have?"

By asking yourself a more empowering question, you regain power. You stop being the victim. You stop being reactive and become proactive. In addition, you'll be surprised at the answers you come up with. They will be answers filled with positivity and perspective.

Whenever you ask yourself a question, you will answer. Our brain is wired to answer questions. It hates open loops and always wants to close them. Even right now, you are asking yourself if what I'm saying is true.

What lie about yourself do you believe? I want to challenge you to confront that lie and replace it with an empowering question that gives you

5

the power. If you'll change your questions, you'll change your life.

Why Most People Fail

I know you may be wondering why I have yet to speak about Intermittent Fasting. I have a reason, trust me.

Yes, I could've started with all the information about intermittent fasting - that's what all the other books do. However, I have to assume that you picked up this book because you have some kind of fitness, dietary, or health goal you are trying to achieve. If that's the case, the best thing I can do is challenge your mindset. It's the ultimate gift. I want to shake your psychology, to push you to get into a mental state where you are forced to succeed.

Tony Robbins says, "80% of success in life is psychology and 20% is mechanics."

I could've jumped straight into the mechanics. But if I didn't challenge your psychology, nothing would change.

I want you to believe this is possible. I want you to commit to the long-term. I want you to focus on process-orientated goals. Above all, I want you to challenge your limiting beliefs and require you to ask empowering questions that will challenge your deepest obstacles.

I hope this chapter has inspired you and allows you to get focused on the task ahead.

CHAPTER 2: INTERMITTENT FASTING: YOUR ULTIMATE WEAPON

Even though intermittent fasting may seem like a new thing, it's not a new thing at all.

In the Paleolithic era our ancestors couldn't wake up, go to the fridge, and make an omelet. They had to go hunt for their food before they could eat. That begs the question - what changed? Well, for the most part we have more convenience now than ever before. It's easy to make breakfast in the morning, so we do. In addition, advertising primarily done by cereal companies have told us that, "Breakfast is the most important meal of the day." This couldn't be further from the truth.

Enter: intermittent fasting (also known as IF).

What is Intermittent Fasting?
"So many people spend their health gaining wealth, and then have to spend their wealth to regain their health." ~ A.J. Materi
In it's simplest form, intermittent fasting is not a diet, but rather a dieting pattern. It functions as a way to schedule your meals so that you get the most out of them. The main concept involves combining periods of eating with periods of not eating. There are several ways to do this, which I'll discuss in the next chapter. Understand though that intermittent fasting doesn't change *what* you eat; it changes *when* you eat.

IF consists of two components: a fasting-window, and an eating-window. Traditionally, during the eating window you have the ability to eat any type of food as long as it falls into within your chosen time frame. Additionally, while no food is allowed during the fasting period, you are allowed to drink water, coffee, tea, and other non-caloric beverages.

When you start intermittent fasting it may be challenging to fast for such a long period of time. However, your body will adapt fairly quickly and it will be become surprisingly simple to do.

Despite what you may think, your energy will not be depleted while doing intermittent fasting. Actually, many people have reported an increase in energy, mental focus, and vitality while doing IF.

Who is This For?
Intermittent fasting can be for everyone. I recommend you consider it if:
- o You are willing to commit.
- o Your partner is supportive.
- o Your job allows for this.

I'd recommend you don't do this if:
- o You are pregnant.
- o You are chronically stressed.
- o You have a history of disordered eating.

Why Intermittent Fasting?
Why should you change the way you're eating?

Intermittent fasting is a great way to lean down without having to do a crazy fat diet or eat 6 tiny meals a day. In fact, most of the time people won't adjust their calories, but cut a meal. Additionally, it has shown to be a great way to keep muscle while getting lean.

Why else?
- o **It works.** Calorie restriction plays a critical role in weight loss. When you fast, you make it easier to restrict your caloric intake over the course of the week. This will give your body the chance to lose weight as you're simply eating less than you were before.

- o **It simplifies your day.** With intermittent fasting, you don't have to prepare, pack, and time your meals out every 3 hours. It gives you the ability to simply skip a meal or two and only worry about your eating window. I'll discuss more benefits in the next chapter.

How Does Intermittent Fasting Work?

You body functions differently when it's in a "fasting" state vs. when it's in a "feasting" state. Whenever you eat a meal, you body spends the next few hours processing the calories. These calories, also known as energy, now enter your bloodstream. Whenever your body needs energy, it will first turn to the energy in your bloodstream instead of the energy stored as fat. This becomes even truer when your body has consumed carbohydrates or sugar, as this is your bodies preferred energy source.

When you are in a fasted state, your body doesn't have all its energy stored in your bloodstream. Therefore, it is required to pull the energy from your fat stores instead of your bloodstream or glycogen in your muscles. This is great for weight loss.

This is also true when working out while "fasted". As the body requires energy, it is unable to pull the required energy from the bloodstream (which is very low because you're in a fasted state), and will turn to your fat stores.

Going deeper:

Studies have shown that your body is most sensitive to insulin during a period of fasting. Whenever you eat, your body reacts by producing insulin. The higher your sensitivity to insulin, the more likely your body will use the food you eat more efficiently. This helps with weight loss and muscle creation.

If you weren't intermediate fasting and chose to eat every couple of hours, your insulin sensitivity would be normal, which would mean your body isn't using the food you eat as effectively. Additionally, when your body needs energy, it will turn to your bloodstream instead of your fat. That's bad for weight loss.

This is why intermittent fasting is one of the best dieting patterns for weight loss.

CHAPTER 3: HOW THIS BENEFITS YOU

Now that you understand *what* intermittent fasting is, let's dive into *how* this benefits you. Here are some of my favorites:

1: Simplicity
- o I love the simplicity intermittent fasting brings. Instead of planning to make breakfast, or thinking through eating 6 small meals everyday, you can just think about two big meals. If you are going out to dinner one night, you can choose to skip breakfast, eat a small lunch, and eat an awesome dinner that evening without ruining your diet.

2: Most Effective Travel Strategy
- o When traveling it can be really hard to stick to your diet. Most restaurants still don't have calorie menus, which make it hard to determine if you are over-eating. However, skipping breakfast and only eating in a certain window will ensure you never over-eat and reverse your results.

3: Easier to Lose Weight
- o If you can get to the point where you are pushing your first meal into the afternoon, you will have a much easier time sticking to your diet. Intermittent fasting allows you to eat bigger meals. These calories are much easier to calculate than 6 smaller meals.

4: Increase Human Growth Hormone
- o This is for those looking to build muscle. With intermittent fasting, your growth hormone in your blood levels may increase as much as 5x. When this happens, it has shown to better facilitate fat burning and muscle gain.

5: Reduced Inflammation and Longer Life Span
o Oxidative stress is one of the causes of aging and many chronic diseases. Intermittent fasting has been shown to decrease oxidative damage and inflammation in the body. This has shown to combat the development of numerous diseases.

6: Brain Function
o When you don't eat for 10-16 hours, your body goes to its fat stores for energy. Fatty acids called ketones are then released into the bloodstream. This has been shown to protect memory, increase learning functionality, and slow disease processes in the brain.

7: Improved Insulin Function
o Insulin is released by our body whenever we consume food and has many roles in regards to metabolism. One of its primary functions is to regulate how the body uses and stores glucose and fat.

o Intermittent fasting has shown to lower insulin levels and increase its sensitivity. Lower levels of insulin, and higher amounts of growth hormone increase the breakdown of body fat and facilitate its use for energy. This has shown to increase metabolism by 3.6-14%, which helps you burn even more calories.

8: Less Diabetes Risk
o Type 2 diabetes has become common in recent years. Its main feature is high blood sugar levels in the context of insulin resistance. Because intermittent fasting helps reduce insulin resistance, it has been shown to lower risks of Type 2 Diabetes.

9: You'll Want Less Food
o Intermittent fasting will help regulate and normalize your gherkin levels. Gherkin is also known as the "hunger hormone".

10: May Help Prevent Cancer
o Cancer is a horrible disease that takes many lives every year. Fasting has been shown to have beneficial effects on the metabolism. This has shown to reduce risk of cancer.

While human studies are needed, there is evidence from animal studies that indicate intermittent fasting may help prevent this deadly disease.

CHAPTER 4: THE BEST INTERMITTENT FASTING METHODS

In this chapter I'm going to show you the best methods for intermittent fasting.

One important note: If you are fasting to lose weight and don't want to count calories, I would encourage you to continue eating as you do right now, but cut out any meals during your fasting window.

An example of this would be to cut out breakfast if you are mainly eating breakfast, lunch, and dinner. This will ensure you are at a caloric deficit, which means you will lose weight. For more advanced strategies and to learn the science behind this, refer to **"Chapter 5: How Fat Loss Works."**

Now, let's talk about some of the different methods of intermittent fasting.

The 16/8 Method (LeanGains)
This method involves fasting every day for 16 hours, and then only eating during an 8 hour "eating window." Martin Berkhan popularized this method, which is known as the LeanGains method.

The method can be very simple. For example, if you were to finish eating dinner around 8pm and you skipped breakfast the next day and only ate at 12PM, you would've effectively followed this method.

This can be hard as your body first adapts. However, once it does you'll be able to breeze through it. One technique I often recommend is to drink coffee in the morning while you are fasting. This helps blunt your appetite, making the fasting easier, and also giving you incredible focus.

Remember that intermittent fasting is a tool, not a magic formula. It's important to note that calories are still important while intermittent fasting. I'd encourage you to still eat healthy during your eating window if you want to see maximum results.

The 5:2 Method
The 5:2 method involves eating normally for 5 days of the week and then restricting your calories to 500-600 on 2 days. It is generally recommended that men restrict themselves to 600, while women restrict themselves to 500.

An example of this would be to eat normally all days of the week except Monday, and Wednesday. Those would be considered your fasting days.

This method is also known as the "fast diet" and was popularized by doctor Michael Mosley.

The 4:3 Method
The 4:3 method functions exactly the same as the 5:2 method. The only added benefit is the diet has an extra calories restricted day, which means you can lose weight faster.

Eat-Stop-Eat
This is a full 24-hour fast, most commonly done 1-2 days a week.

When you choose to fast with Eat-Stop-Eat doesn't really matter. You can finish dinner on a Monday night at 6PM and decide to fast to a 6PM dinner the following night. That will complete the 24-hour period. You can choose to do a lunch-to-lunch fast, or a breakfast-to-breakfast fast – it's truly up to you.

If you choose to do this, don't feel pressured to jump in right away. 24 hours is a long time. Feel free to start slow. As an example, you can start with a full 16-hour fast and then slowly build up.

Remember, during your eating period it is imperative that you do not eat more than you usually would. After 24 hours, some people are so hungry that they overeat and undo the progress they made. This will lead to little or no results.

Alternate-Day

Alternate-Day fasting is for hardcore intermittent fasters. The basic idea is that you would fast every second day. There are various methods, some of which are a full 24-hour fast, while others limit calories to 500 during fasting days.

If you are just starting out, I'd recommend you skip this alternate-day fasting and choose another method.

Warrior Diet

The Warrior Diet, popularized by Ori Hofmekler, involves eating small amounts of vegetables and raw fruits throughout the day and then eating a huge meal in the evening.

The food choices during the Warrior Diet most resemble that of the Paleo diet. They are whole, unprocessed foods that look similar to how they appear in nature.

A lot of people enjoy this as they are able to continually snack throughout the day and never have to deal with the feeling of intense hunger.

Spontaneous Meal Skipping

For some, this is the easiest method and still works well. Spontaneous meal skipping involves fasting through a specific meal during the day.

If you're anything like me, I can often forget about a meal because I'm so busy at work. Spontaneous meal skipping encourages not making up for that meal but instead fasting until the next one.

CHAPTER 5: HOW FAT LOSS WORKS

To understand how fat loss works, you need to have a firm understanding of two things:
- Calories
- Total Daily Energy Expenditure (Abbreviated as TDEE. I'll also refer to this as maintenance calories, or homeostasis)

Understanding Calories & TDEE

To put it in the simplest terms, calories are energy. When we eat, we consume calories. As we move, exercise, and breathe we burn calories.

Calories are a way of keeping track of your body's energy budget. We achieve a healthy balance when we put in as many calories as we burn. When we consistently consume more calories than we burn the body will store the excess energy as fat. This will lead to us picking up weight. When we consume fewer calories than we burn, the body converts the excess fat in our bodies into energy and uses that to meet its demands.

In more literal terms, a calorie is the energy it would take to raise 1 kilogram of water by 1 degree Celsius.

Everything that we eat contains calories. These calories tell us the energy that is stored in an item of food's chemical bonds. When we eat it, that energy is released through digestion.

Calories are used in three areas. 10% is used for digestion, 20% is used for physical activity, and 70% for the bodies basic organs and tissues. That 70% corresponds with what is known as your Basil Metabolic Rate (BMR). Your BMR is the amount of calories your body needs to keep you alive if you eat nothing, and did nothing all day.

Add digestion and physical activity back into the mix, and you have what is known as your Total Daily Energy Expenditure (TDEE). This is a measurement of the amount of calories a person needs each day. We will also refer to this as your maintenance calories (the amount of calories you need for your weight to stay exactly the same).

The average guidelines for TDEE are 2,000 calories for woman, and 2,500 calories for men (which is based on average weight, age, muscle mass, and physical activity). The average guidelines for BMR are 1,400 for women, and 1,750 for men. One caveat is that your BMR can be down-regulated, or up-regulated depending on your eating patterns – more on that later.

Does that mean every guy can eat for 2,500 calories? Probably not. If you were running a marathon, the average person would burn 2,600 calories. This means that if an average guy with a BMR of 1,750 ran a marathon and burned 2,600, they would need to consume 4,350 calories to maintain weight for that day.

One thing to note is that top of all of this; there are some factors that can alter BMR. These factors are things like intestine length, gut bacteria, enzyme levels, and thyroid functionality. All of these variables can alter the way different people extract energy from food. If you're concerned that one of these variables could affect you, be sure to consult a doctor.

Hopefully you're still with me. We just got through the most complicated part, I promise.

Weight Loss/Gain Formulas
Weight loss in itself is a pretty simple concept. I know that may sound weird, especially because of all the confusion in the fitness community. However, it can be brought down to a simple formula:

1: Weight Loss Formula = Eating less than you burn.
o   OR Calories < Burn = Weight Loss
2: Weight Gain Formula = Eating more than you burn.
o   OR Calories > Burn = Weight Gain

If you follow the weight loss formula, you will lose fat. If you follow the weight gain formula, you will pick up fat (unless you are on a strength training program). It's that easy.

Note: there are some people/articles out there that will disagree with me. However, most professionals agree that this is the fact. Additionally, in my personal experience, I have seen these formulas work every time.

How Do I Know How Many Calories are in Food?

All foods have what are called macronutrients. These macronutrients are protein, carbohydrates, and fat. They all serve specific functions (Which is one reason why I don't like fad diets that require you to cut any of these).

Protein: Simply put, protein is your building block of muscle. They work in the cells and are required for structure, function, and regulation of the body's organs and tissues.
- o When it comes to food, every gram of protein converts to 4 calories.
- o A few good sources of protein are: chicken, salmon, and whole eggs.

Fats: Contrary to popular belief, fats aren't something to be feared. Fats are essential to a healthy diet as they improve brain development, overall cell functioning, and protect your body's organs.
- o When it comes to food, every gram of fat converts to 9 calories.
- o A few good sources of fats are: almonds, walnuts, avocados, and olives.

Carbohydrates: Carbohydrates are comprised of sugar, starch, and fibers, which our body breaks down into glucose and uses for energy. They are our body's primary source of energy.
- o When it comes to food, every gram of carbohydrates converts to 4 calories.
- o A few good sources of carbohydrates are: fruits (apples, bananas), vegetables (broccoli, sweet potatoes), and whole grains (brown rice, oats).

Calories in a Pound of Fat/Muscle

Fat: There are approximately 3,500 calories in a pound of fat. That means that for every 3,500 calories that you eat over your maintenance calories (or TDEE), you will pick up 1 pound of fat.

The inverse of this is also true. Every time you eat 3,500 less than your maintenance calories, you lose 1 pound of fat.

Muscle: There are approximately 2,500 calories in a pound of muscle. Under great conditions, the average person on an intense strength based workout plan can pick up half a pound of lean muscle per week. That means in order to give your body the calories needed to gain muscle, you should eat an excess of 1,250 calories over maintenance during a week to gain muscle. This works out to be about 180 calories a day above maintenance.

A Quick Story: I remember talking to my friend a few months ago. At the time, he was trying to pick up weight but couldn't and was feeling demotivated. He told me that he couldn't gain weight because his metabolism was too quick. You may have heard a statement like this before. I want you to understand the reality.

Our bodies are always trying to achieve homeostasis (balance) and when we eat more, our bodies attempt to up-regulate our metabolisms to get there. When we eat less, our bodies attempt to down-regulate.

For my friend struggling to gain weight, it simply means one these two things are true:
1. His BMR (basil metabolic rate) is high because he has trained it to be so. If this is the case, he needs to start eating more than he currently is to pick up weight.
2. His TDEE (BMR + daily activity) is incredibly high and he is burning more than he is eating.

With my friend, I started by asking a few questions about his daily habits. I realized his job requires him to be on his feet all day (think: doctor, nurse, construction worker etc.). Because he is on his feet all day, his daily activity is insanely high (much higher than someone who sits at a desk all day). That means he needs to either move less or eat more to pick up weight.

Because moving less isn't an option for him, I advised him to start eating 500 calories more than he was. As he started tracking his intake and eating more, he was able to start picking up weight.

Putting It All Together
I hope this chapter has brought understanding to how fat loss and weight gain can occur. I tried to make it as simple as possible. My goal is to give you a clear understanding so that *you* have the ability to decide how to go about losing/gaining weight. You understand your body better than anyone else. Which means, the power is truly in your hands.

In the next chapter, we are going to put together everything we've learned so far to create a personalized plan just for you.

Enjoying the book so far? If so, I would love for you to leave a review on Amazon. This will help this book can get into as many hands as possible. There are people just like you who need help. Reviewing the book will help get the word out.

Go here to leave a review: http://amzn.to/2lt7v5c

I also welcome your feedback! If you have any suggestions on how to improve the book, please contact me: noahlively.ebooks@publishingwhale.com

CHAPTER 6: POWERFUL PROTOCOLS

In this chapter, I have listed two categories of protocols. One category relates to your mental performance, while the other relates to nutrition. Whether or not you choose to do the mental performance protocol is up to you. However, I do recommend that you pick one of the nutrition protocols that aligns most with your goals.

Mental Performance Protocol

I've mentioned this in part already, but it's too powerful not to talk through again. One of the main goals and benefits of intermittent fasting is the intense level of focus you will feel. When everyone at your office goes out to lunch and blows their meal plan (and budget), they get a massive insulin spike which results in a massive crash later. While they are struggling to get their focus back, you will be fasted and as focused as ever. That's why intermittent fasting can truly change the way you work and increase your performance.

Here is the protocol:

1: Drink caffeine first thing in the morning.

In order to achieve the best benefits, I recommend that you drink coffee or green tea first thing in the morning. The caffeine will suppress your appetite, wake you up, and help you focus. Additionally, caffeine has been shown to boost memory; increase reaction time and logical reasoning; and reduce chronic inflammation.

2: Drink a second cup when you start to feel hungry again.

This will help you push your fast late into the day. However, be careful not to drink caffeine after 2pm as it may affect your sleep.

3: Push your first meal to after 2pm.

This will help you to keep focus for most of the day because your body is focused on the task at hand and not digesting your food. I would recommend a packed lunch that doesn't have carbs that are high on the glycemic index - think brown rice, vegetables, sweet potatoes, etc.

If you get hungry before 2pm, I recommend you eat an apple, which only has 100 calories and will restore your glycogen to make you feel full.

If you choose to implement the mental performance protocol you will find that you will be able to focus through the majority of your workday. This will help you be fully present and ensure that you are a top performer. As an added benefit, it will save you cash from going out to eat too.

Structuring Your Diet

Before we jump into the nutrition protocol, I want you to understand how we will structure your diet. Our goal would be to structure it for maximum muscle and minimum fat.

To maximize muscle growth / minimize fat gain we need to ensure that these three things are true:

1. You are providing your body with enough calories to support either gaining muscle or losing fat.
2. You are taking in optimum amounts of protein, fats, and carbs to best support your goals.
3. You are taking in optimum vitamins and minerals to promote recovery and health.

Macro Nutrients: Proteins, Fat, Carbs

In order to have the best results, we must consume optimum macro nutrient amounts to support a healthy lifestyle. This is applicable whether your goal is to build muscle or lose fat.

Protein: Most people think you need to eat an insane amount of protein to gain muscle, however this isn't necessarily true. In fact, .82g of protein per pound of body weight seems to be the optimum amount of protein for muscle building.

However, just to be safe, I often recommend eating around 1g per pound of body weight. For example, if you weighed 180 pounds, you would eat 180g of protein.

Fats: As I mentioned in the previous chapter, fat is critical to hormone function and also plays a key role in testosterone. For this reason, I would recommend getting about 30% of your calories from fat.

Carbohydrates: Carbohydrates are what the body uses most often for energy. We will use carbohydrates to meet the remainder of your caloric budget.

In order to get a good amount of vitamins, I recommend that you include foods such as broccoli, asparagus, and spinach in your diet where possible.

Nutrition Protocols
Read through the following nutrition protocols and pick the one that most aligns with your goals.

Extreme Weight Loss Protocol
Use this if: You want to lose a lot of weight fast.

Calculating a calorie budget:
The extreme weight loss protocol will ensure that you are losing weight incredibly quickly. Results will typically be in the range of 1-2 pounds per week if you are between 10-15% body fat. If your body fat is higher than this, results can be more substantial.

This is how you would calculate your daily calorie budget: take your goal weight and multiply it by 10.

This is applicable for both women and men. For instance, if you are a 200-pound male and you would like to weigh 180 pounds, then you will eat 180 x 10 = 1,800 calories. This will ensure you are losing weight at an incredibly fast rate. Also, because you are intermittent fasting, eating 1,800 calories is a lot easier because you don't have to split that into 6 small meals.

Now, let me show you how the math works.

An average 180-pound male would have a TDEE (maintenance calories budget) of around 2,500-2,800 (For the sake of this illustration, let's use a maintenance budget of about 2,650 calories). That means if this man ate 2,650 calories every day, he would maintain his weight.

If this man's goal is to weigh 180 pounds, he would eat 1,800 calories (180 x 10 = 1,800 calories). This is a daily calorie deficit of 850 calories (2,650 maintenance calorie budget - 1,800 calories eaten = 850 deficit).

Remember how I said there are 3,500 calories in a pound of fat?

An 850-calorie deficit multiplied over 7 days would equal a 5,950-calorie deficit. This would equal a loss of 1.7 pounds of body fat in a week (5,950 calories divided by 3,500 calories in a pound of body fat = 1.7).

Note: You should only do the extreme weight loss protocol for 8 weeks at a time. As you eat at a deficit, your metabolism can down-regulate. If you lose weight initially and it stalls, this shows that your body has adjusted (reached homeostasis). If this is the case, look at the section on **"Reverse Dieting"** below to rebuild your metabolism. When your metabolism is back up to normal, you can enter another fat loss phase.

If you find that you have already been eating according to the extreme weight loss protocol for the past few months and have stopped losing weight, then consult the **"Reverse Dieting"** section below.

Lean Bulk Protocol
Use this if: You are happy with your fat levels and want to build lean muscle.

Traditional bulking is largely ineffective. It requires people to pick up a large amount of weight, which is mostly fat. Often people are able to gain far during in the bulk, but not lose it after. This is because, from a psychological view, bulking is always easier than cutting. By doing a "lean bulk" we ensure this doesn't happen.

The lean bulk protocol is for those who want to pack on some good muscle without having to do the traditional (and ineffective) bulk and cut cycles. Lean bulking is a protocol used by professionals all around the world to ensure that they are always looking their best while gaining muscle – so no more cutting down for vacation or being caught of guard.

Calculating maintenance calories:
In order to do a lean bulk, we need to calculate your maintenance calories. To accomplish this, you can use a **TDEE calculator** on the Internet.

However, it's important to note that these calculators are known to over-estimate the amount of calories you can really need. Following this overestimation can lead to fat-gain.

A second method, my recommendation, is your body weight x 14-16. Use a 14 multiplier if you tend to gain weight easily, use a 16 multiplier if it's harder for you to pick up fat, and use a 15 multiplier if you feel like you're in the middle. For women, I recommend starting with a 14 multiplier.

For example, if you are a 180-pound male who gains weight rather quickly, you would calculate 180 pounds x 14 = 2,520. In this case, 2,520 would be your predicted maintenance calories.

Now, the sweet spot to making this a "lean bulk" is to add about 180 calories per day above maintenance. This will ensure that you support your body with the calories it needs to build muscle.

How did I get to that number? There is roughly 2,500 calories in a pound of muscle. In the best circumstances, someone can pick up about half a pound of muscle per week, which is about 1,250 calories. 1,250 calories divided by 7 days = 179 calories.

If you follow this protocol and find that your waist measurements are going up, reduce your calories by about 50-100 per day. Again, this is totally dependent on how your body responds. Ideally, you want to get into a place where week-by-week your weight is going up, but your waist measurements stay the same or only go up a little. This will ensure that your weight gain is from muscle, not fat.

Also, only try a lean bulk protocol when combined with a muscle-building program. If you aren't trying to build muscle, the excess calories will be turned to fat.

Recomposition Protocol
Use this if: You want continue building muscle, and lose fat at a slower rate.

The recomposition protocol is going to help you build muscle, while losing a little fat every week. I recommend that you eat at a calorie surplus on training days, and at a calorie deficit on rest days when doing the recomposition protocol.

Calculating Recomposition Protocol Calorie Budget

1: Calculate your maintenance calories. If you don't know how to do this yet, refer to the **"calculating maintenance calories"** under the **"lean bulk protocol"**.

Once you have your maintenance calories you can move onto step 2.

2: Calculate your calorie budget. As an example, let's say you were a 180-pound guy, whose maintenance calories are 2,500, when training 4 times a week. In this case, your calories would be the following.

o   On rest days (3x a week) = eat 400 *under* maintenance
o   On training days (4x a week) = eat 300 *over* maintenance.

This would respectively equate to weekly calorie surplus of 0.

That means if maintenance was 2,500 calories, you would eat 2,100 calories on rest days, and 2,800 calories on training days.

Reverse Dieting Protocol
Use this if:

o   You are eating very little (under 1,500) but aren't losing weight.
o   You want to increase your metabolic rate and enter an active fat loss period at a later stage.

Your body's main goal is to try and keep you alive. This is an incredible function but unfortunately can also make fat loss stall. Allow me to illustrate…

Imagine we lived like cavemen. Every morning we would need to wake up and go hunt for food. If we were unsuccessful, we would in essence starve.

When our bodies realize we are starving, it shuts down various functions and will down regulate our metabolism in order to keep us alive for longer. Our bodies can't tell the difference between trying to lose weight and being in a famine.

This is something I've seen countless of times. People can be eating next to nothing and still not losing weight. If you are experiencing this, then you need to go into a reverse dieting phase to correct your metabolism.

The reverse dieting protocol is essentially a tool that will allow you to up-regulate your metabolism. Once your metabolism has returned to normal (eating 1800-2500 calories for women and 2000-2800 for men, but not picking up fat), you can enter another fat loss phase.

One word of caution, reverse dieting is *very* specific and requires a high level of commitment. If you aren't very careful, this can lead to fat gain. But if done correctly, it will give you incredible results. I know some people that have even lost weight while doing this. Your results will be totally dependent on your natural body composition and how closely you follow the protocol.

The science behind it:

Imagine you were eating 2,500 calories and maintaining weight. Then, you decided to cut your calories to 1,500. You would experience massive fat loss initially (about 2 pounds per week). Eventually, your body would adjust to that amount of calories and you would stop losing weight. When this happens, most people continue cutting their calories.

Let's imagine that after a few months, you were now eating 1,000 calories. Your body has, yet again, readjusted and achieved homeostasis (equilibrium) and you aren't losing weight. This is where most people mess up their results. During this stage, if you were to go out with your friends and eat a dinner that was 2,000 calories, your body would effectively take 1,000 calories and store it as fat. It's a bit more complicated in that, but let's keep it there for now to make it simple.

While this all sounds wrong, it isn't. Your body is simply trying to keep you alive in this "perceived famine."

After that one night out with your friends, your weight will go up. Most people freak out when they see that and cut their calories back down to 1,000. This will create the yo-yo diet effect that you have often heard about:
  o   We eat very little. We achieve homeostasis.
  o   We binge eat, or eat too much. We pick up fat.
  o   We freak out, and go back to eating very little. We again achieve homeostasis.
  o   We eat too much. We pick up fat.
  o   The cycle continues.

Reverse dieting is the only effective way to break this when you are eating so little.

I so wish I could get this information in front of everyone. I know girls who have been eating 600 calories a day and walk around so discouraged about their progress. Unable to lose weight, they think they are broken. That's

27

not the case. This protocol will help.

Next, I'll show you how this is done.

How to Reverse Diet
Day 1:
Step 1: Determine the current calories you are eating on a daily basis. Use a food calculator (**myfitnesspal**, and **netmydiary** are great solutions) and track *all* your calories for a normal day. This would be your starting point. Let's say your average calories are 1,500.

Day 2:
Step 1: Determine your macro targets. First, set your protein consumption for 1g of protein per pound of body weight. If you weighed 140, then you set your protein for 140g per day.

Step 2: Subtract your protein calories from your current calorie budget.
- o 140g of protein x 4 calories per gram = 560 calories from protein.
- o 1,500 total calories - 560 calories from protein = 940 calories remaining.

Step 3: Split your remaining calories by carbohydrates and fat. Give 60% to carbohydrates, and 40% to fat. Let's start with calculating the percentages:
- o 940 remain calories x .6 (60% carbs) = 564 calories from carbs
- o 940 remain calories x .4 (40% fats) = 376 calories from fats.

Next, let's calculate how many grams of carbs and fats that would equate to:
- o 564 calories from carbs / 4 calories per gram = 141g of carbs.
- o 376 calories from fats / 9 calories per gram = 42g of fat.

You now have your baseline macro targets. Technically, if you did the math I showed you and kept eating this many calories, your weight should stay the same. But you may lose or gain a little initially until your metabolism balances.

Step 4: Determine how quickly you will increase your carbs and fats on a weekly level. A few things to consider:
- o If you increase really quickly, you may pick up more fat. However, if you care more about eating normally than gaining fat, I would suggest speeding up the process a bit.
- o If you plan on weight training, you can be a bit more aggressive in bringing up your calories. Weight lifting is shown to slow down some

of the fat gain associated with reverse dieting.
- o If you have a history of binge eating or breaking your diet, I would recommend that you are aggressive with bringing up your calories quickly. This might lead to initial weight gain, but will negate the yoyo effect.

Step 5: Decide 3 days of the week that you will weigh yourself and/or take your stomach measurements. This will help measure your progress.
- o Remember, the scale is a *tool* and not a measurement of your *worth*. People often allow the number on a scale to scare them. It is completely normal for your weight to fluctuate 0-2 pounds a day. So don't get too wrapped up in it.

Step 6: Decide your reverse dieting speed.
- o For aggressive reverse dieters: Take your carbs and fats up by about 6-10% every week. We have already optimized your protein so that wouldn't need to be adjusted.

- o For conservative reverse dieters: Take your carbs and fats up by about 2-5% every week.

- o If you find that you've added 5% to your calories and you aren't picking up weight, this shows you are adapting well. In this case, you can start to be more aggressive.

If after a 2-5% increase you are picking up weight dramatically, I would encourage you to *not* adjust anything. People tend to freak out and drop their calories back to where they started. But this increases the yoyo effect. The best thing you can do is continue eating the same amount and eventually your metabolism will level out. Once it does, continue increasing your calories by smaller percentages (Around 2%-3% depending on how well you are adapting).

What to do after my reverse diet?
After a few weeks/months of doing this you will find that you are able to eat substantially more while still maintaining your weight. Congratulations, you have just up-regulated your metabolism. At this point you can decide to:
- o **1: Continue reverse dieting.** To do this, keep increasing your calories until you have reached the upper threshold of your metabolic ability. The higher you can take this, the easier it would be for you to build muscle and diet in the future.
- o **2: Maintain your weight.** To do this, simply stop adding calories and continue to eat the same calories / macros.

o **3: Enter a fat loss phase.** To do this, lower your calories. You can do an aggressive approach like the "Extreme Weight Loss Protocol", or you can take a more controlled approach. If you would like to do a more controlled approach, lower your daily calories by 250-500. At this rate you would lose 1/2 - 1 pound a week. Whenever your weight loss stalls, lower your calories by another 250-500 (Note: I recommend that you never lower your calories below 1,200 without consulting a professional).

How to Optimize Your Results

Through all of this, I want to encourage you to keep track of your weight and measurements. Choose a day when you can do a weekly weigh in. I'd suggest starting with Saturday mornings.

After you wake up and use the bathroom, weigh yourself when fully undressed and take your measurements. Keep track of these and compare to the next week's results.

If you find that you are picking up weight and your waist measurement is staying the same, you are building muscle. Keep going.

If you find that your waist measurement is going up, that's a sign you are eating too much. Dial back your calories by 100 calories (unless you are on the reverse diet protocol. In which case, keep your calories the same until you reach homeostasis). Keep doing this until you have found your maintenance calories.

This is the most effective way to determine your *actual* maintenance calories. By tracking your weight gain/loss every week, you will be more effective than a fitness device or a calculator on the Internet. This is most effective because you are measuring your progress by actual *results*, and not just some formula.

After you have done your measurements, take progress pictures. Take a relaxed front, side, and back pose. I recommend that you download the app **"Layout"** (Or a similar picture stitching/collage app), and then an app like **"Over"** that will allow you to place text over the picture.

Create a collage of the three poses, date the picture, and store it in a folder on your phone. This will give you easy access to visible progress from week to week, which is critical for motivation. It will also give you some great before and after images with the timeline to be able to share your fitness journey with others.

Common Questions

1: What do I do if I have been eating well below maintenance calories and I have stopped losing weight?

o This probably means that your metabolism has adjusted to your level of intake. If this is the case, lower your calories if you are still in a healthy zone (1,300+ calories for women, 1,600+ calories for men). If you were a woman eating below 1,200 calories or a man eating below 1,500 calories, I would recommend that you **reverse diet**, bring your calories back up over a few weeks (strengthen your metabolism), and then start dieting again.

2: I think I have damaged my metabolism. What should I do?

It is highly unlikely that your metabolism is "damaged." Our bodies are incredibly adaptable which means they have the ability to survive on very few calories.

While metabolic damage doesn't occur, metabolic adaption does. If your body can be adapted down, it can be adapted up. Newton hit the nail on the head with his third law, "For every action, there is an equal and opposite reaction."

Take a deep breath. You're ok. Don't read crazy online articles that try to sell you some magic pill to "fix your broken metabolism." Read the **reverse dieting section** and you will be able to build your metabolism back up to normal.

CHAPTER 7: BUILDING MUSCLE WITH INTERMITTENT FASTING

Welcome to the chapter on building muscle. In this chapter, I hope to debunk muscle-building myths and show you how building muscle works.

Muscles Building Overview

Muscles are the "engines" our bodies use to propel itself. There is a direct correlation to the way we treat our muscles and the way we grow our muscles.

Every time you are about to lift an object, your brain sends a signal to motor neurons in our limbs (arms, legs, etc.). These motor neurons fire once they receive the signal. This causes certain muscles to relax and others to contract. For example, if you were picking up a cup of coffee your bicep would contract, but your triceps would relax. This is what allows you to pick up the object.

The larger the challenge, the larger the signal to the brain. The larger the signal to the brain, the more motor neurons are fired.

Whenever you place your muscles under more stress than they are used to, the cells experience microscopic damage. These damaged cells release cytokines, an inflammatory molecule, which activates the immune system to repair the damage. This repair process is muscle growth.

The greater the damage, the greater the need for repair.

People often ask, "So doesn't that mean I can lift a small rock and build muscle?"

The answer is, no not necessarily. Because our muscles have already adapted to every day tasks, these don't place the amount of stress needed to build muscle (also called hypertrophy).

In order to access hypertrophy and build muscle, you must expose your muscles to a higher volume than they are used to. When you do this, in combination with adequate nutrition and rest, your muscles will grow. If you stop exposing your muscles to these higher tensions, they will shrink. This is a process known as muscle atrophy.

All this is why protein is so important. Protein is the building block for muscle as it preserves our muscle mass in the form of amino acids. Amino acids are used to repair our muscle, therefore making it critical for building muscle.

Like I said before, our bodies are continually adapting. If you continue to place your muscles under new stress, eat right, rest, and repeat - you will create the conditions necessary to build muscle.

Common Terms to Know

1: Strength Training: Strength Training (or weight lifting) is by far the most effective way to build muscle. Historically, humans with the highest muscular development are all weight lifters.

2: Volume: If you've ever looked at the largest natural body builder next to the largest natural power lifter, you will notice that body builders have more muscular development than power lifters.

This is mostly because of the volume difference in their training. Body builders tend to train in much higher total volume than a power lifter who is training for the highest weight possible. Volume is determined by the following equation:
- o   Amount of sets x number of repetitions x weight lifted.
- o   Or to put it more simply: Volume = Sets x Reps x Weight.

Volume is effective because as you increase volume, you place new stress on the muscle, which causes growth.

3: Intensity: If you've been in the body building game for a while, you will know about something called your 1 rep maximum (1RM). This is a unit of measurement that indicates the total weight you are capable of lifting for 1 full repetition. Intensity is defined as the percent value of that 1 rep maximum.

4: Failure: Most of the time when training, you want to push your muscles to "failure." Failure happens when you are unable to complete the rep. In most cases, failure is lifting a weight to half motion but "failing" to complete the full range of motion for the exercise. Generally, when you reach failure, the set is complete.

Failure ensures that you have sufficiently exhausted the muscle and recruited all it's muscle fibers. Often, training to failure ensures you have given a set everything you've got so that with adequate nutrition, you can come back stronger next time.

Note: I generally recommend all beginner lifters train to failure. However, I want you to understand failure is a tool, not a rule. Allow me to explain. Failure ensures you are pushing yourself to your max, which is great. However, reaching failure for every set can also can be incredibly tiring. Some people are able to achieve more volume by achieving failure for every set, while others can achieve more volume by stopping one rep short of failure and saving energy for the next set.

You simply need to experiment what works best for you. Your ultimate exercise outcome for building muscle should be to do more volume today than you did before. If you achieve that outcome through failure, continue doing it. If you achieve that outcome through stopping one rep short, continue doing that. If you find failure on biceps allows for more volume than failure on chest, then push biceps to failure.

The bottom line is this: Fitness is incredibly unique to each individual. Find what works for you, and continue doing that. I hope that's helpful.

How Muscle is Built
Let's go a bit further with protein. Protein in muscle is no different to protein found in food. These are long chains of amino acids that have attached to one another in the skeletal muscle. The question is how does this process work?

There are two competing processes that determine muscle mass.
1. **Protein synthesis** (the act of attaching amino acids to one another and making them into muscle).
2. **Protein breakdown** (the act of various specialty enzymes that cleave off amino acids in the muscle).

34

These are normal processes. The body is in a continuum of breaking down and rebuilding tissue in the body. It allows our bodies to adapt to the demands that are placed on it and remodel itself based on the signal it receives.

Muscle building depends on the balancing of protein synthesis and protein breakdown.
- If protein synthesis *exceeds* protein breakdown, your muscle mass will increase.
- If protein synthesis *equals* protein breakdown, you will have no change in muscle mass.
- If protein synthesis *is less than* protein breakdown, your muscle mass decreases.

In order to build bigger muscles, you need to increase protein synthesis, decrease protein breakdown, or both.

The challenge is that building muscle not only increases protein synthesis, it also increases protein breakdown. This shows the bodies ability to adapt like I said earlier.

Whenever we force a muscle to contract against a heavy load, the primary response is protein synthesis. Protein synthesis will occur 24-48 hours after the muscles are strained. If we have adequate nutrition during that period, the muscle will grow. If we don't have the adequate nutrition, the body will breakdown another muscle to repair the broken one. The other factor is protein breakdown. Insulin from carbs actually inhibits protein breakdown. Which is why including carbs in your diet is so important after all. [1]

Let's get a bit geekier. Mammalian Target of Rapamycin, or mTOR for short, is a master controller of protein synthesis. There is a direct connection between muscle growth and mTOR activation. The more a workout activates mTOR, the more protein synthesis happens. Three things activate mTOR:
- Mechanical stress (which happens from training heavy loads)
- Growth factors (IFG-1, growth hormone, insulin)
- Amino acids

What does all this mean? If you lift heavy (activating mTOR and protein synthesis), eat protein at some point during the day (creating the building blocks for muscle and protein synthesis), and eat carbs (releasing insulin that inhibits protein breakdown), your muscles will grow.

What is the Primary Stimulus for Growth?
1: Progressive Overload:

Progressive overload has been considered by many to be the most important principle behind muscle building. Progressive overload involves increasing the weight, repetition, and sets of your exercises. Done right, you will be able to get stronger and continuously lift heavier weight than previously. This will continue to place the muscle under new stress that will cause it to tear, which with the right nutrition and rest will cause it to grow.

In order to achieve progressive overload, it is important that you use a progression model. A progression model is a strategy that determines when to add more volume. I recommend using a weight that will allow you to fail in the given rep range. Continue pushing yourself every week. When you are able to exceed the suggested rep range, increase the weight of that set by 5 pounds. If you find you are unable to increase the weight, you can substitute it for an additional set.

Here's an example of what it might look like to increase your weight every week. Imagine you were benching 185. You were on your 4th set which requires you to do between 4-6 reps.
- o   Week 1: 185x4 (achieved failure)
- o   Week 2: 185x5 (achieved failure; added a rep)
- o   Week 3: 185x6 (achieved failure; added a rep)
- o   Week 4: 185x7 (achieved failure; surpassed rep range of 4-6)
- o   Week 5: 190x4 (achieved failure; added 5 pounds)
- o   Week 6: 190x5 (achieved failure; added a rep)
- o   Etc.

Whenever your reps exceed the given rep range, as seen in week 4 of our example, the following week you will take your weight up by 5 pounds and lift to failure. Then continue to do this for all your sets.

Training Philosophy

The training programs set out in this book will train you within all the known rep ranges that cause muscle growth. These programs have been optimized to ensure you have:
- o   A lot of volume
- o   Progressive overload
- o   Achieved failure

These 3 components will ensure you will build muscle in the most efficient way possible.

Our reps will range from 1-20 reps. Rep range is a topic with many differing opinions. Some people recommend 8-12, while others recommend 4-6, and others recommend 15+. There are enough articles on this idea alone to fill up multiple encyclopedias.

With this kind of debate, I tend to look to what both scientists and body builders have discovered. One recent controlled study showed that higher reps vs. lower reps didn't have a drastic enough statistical difference to say which one is better.

Here's the truth, as long as all sets are pushed to the limit and volume is increased, the results will work. Period.

With that said, this is why I like higher volume. Higher volume ensures:
1. **You get a pump**. While most people think of a "pump" as a short-term cosmetic effect, it can actually result in greater muscle development. Studies have shown that cellular swelling, which is caused by a pump, increase both protein synthesis and decrease protein breakdown. If you paid attention before, you know that's good. Getting a pump is really hard to do with lower level of reps.

2. **Maximized time under tension.** Not only will you be lifting a larger amount of weight with high volume training, (placing your body under more stress) but, because of the length of the sets, you will be under tension for longer.

3. **Getting higher reps to failure.** Higher reps require more eccentric contractions, which have been shown to create more muscular damage. There is a lot of evidence that suggests that muscular damage and hypertrophy (muscle growth) are linked.

Building Muscle While Intermittent Fasting
Is it possible to build muscle while intermittently fasting? Absolutely!

I was able to put on lean muscle quite easily while following intermittent fasting. Remember, you will gain muscle as long as you are eating above your maintenance calorie level, eating the right macronutrients, resting, and strength-training consistently.

I recommend you follow the **lean bulk**, **recomposition**, or **reverse dieting protocol** (depending on your goals) and you will be able to pick up lean muscle.

Losing Weight & Building Muscle Simultaneously

When it comes to losing weight and building muscle, it is a little more complicated. Remember that I said losing weight happens when you eat *less* than your maintenance calories and building muscle happens when you eat a little *more* than your maintenance calories. From a purely nutritional standpoint, it is impossible to do both.

There is one small caveat. From what I've seen in studies and my personal experience, losing weight while building muscle is easy for someone who has just started weight training. When someone is just starting out, their muscles aren't used to any form of excess stress. Beginner lifters will be able to experience rapid strength gains, which in turn will lead to muscle growth, even if they are eating at a deficit.

If you are a more advanced lifter, your muscles have adapted to stress, making it harder to put on additional muscle. At an advanced level, most people who try building muscle while eating at a deficit experience a decline in their strength. When your strength or volume goes down, your muscles will go through atrophy. When you aren't using your muscle fibers, your body adapts, energy can be taken from your muscle, and they will get smaller.

That's why I recommend advanced lifters choose to either build muscle or lose fat at any given time.

CHAPTER 8: EXERCISE PLAN

While exercise isn't directly a part of intermittent fasting, it is critical to a healthy lifestyle.

Because everyone has different goals, I have broken this section up into two approaches: cardio and weight lifting. At the end of this chapter, I'll help you choose the one that is most appropriate for you. You may also choose to combine both exercise approaches for optimal benefits.

Exercise Approach
Cardio:
When doing cardio for fat loss, you want to look at various aerobic activities. There are a number of different exercises you can do for cardio. Any one of these exercises will ensure that you are burning additional fat. You can choose your intensity level based on your goals.

1: Walking (Burns roughly 300-400 calories per hour): Walking is great for both beginners and those that have been previously injured. However, walking has a much lower intensity than some other cardio exercises.
   o   Suggested frequency: 3-6 times a week.
   o   Duration: 20-45 minutes per session.

2: Running (Burns roughly 600 calories per hour):
Because running requires a higher intensity than walking, you will burn calories quicker. Running is considered a rather high impact exercise and can hurt your joints over time if you aren't careful.
   o   Suggested frequency: 3-6 times a week.

o   Duration: 20-30m per session.

3: Cycling (Burns around 600 calories per hour):
Cycling, in a similar manner to running, involves all the same muscles with a much lower impact on your joints. This makes it an ideal way to train for virtually anyone.
o   Suggested frequency: 3-6 times a week.
o   Duration: 20-30m per session.

4: Rowing (Burns around 840 calories per hour):
This is my personal favorite cardio exercise. Rowing is a total body workout and uses all your muscles. It has high intensity, burning more calories per hour than any other commonly used aerobic exercise, and has incredibly low impact on your joints.
o   Suggested frequency: 3-6 times a week.
o   Duration: 30-45m per session.

5: Jumping Rope (Burns over 1000 calories per hour):
Jumping rope is a very high impact activity but provides an incredible workout when performed correctly. It has an added bonus of being very portable, affordable, and can even be done indoors. Jumping rope is also a great way to add muscle definition to your calves and shoulders. It's not quite as easy as it looks, but once you get the hang of it, the results are well worth the effort.
o   Suggested frequency: 3-6 times a week.
o   Duration: 15-45m per session.

6: Yoga (Burns 200-600 calories per hour):
Yoga is an incredibly low impact activity which increases flexibility, muscle strength and tone. In addition, yoga can be done from the comfort of your own home and is known to help respiration, energy, and vitality. My friend **Zoe Bray-Cotton** has put together a course which I highly recommend if you're ready to give yoga a try.
• Suggested program: **Yoga Burn for women**.

Weight Lifting:
When it comes to weight lifting, I strongly recommend that you try volume training. During this type of training, you will sufficiently exhaust the muscles, access all your muscle fibers, and increase mass and strength. I recommend training at least 5 days a week. If this is not possible with your schedule, you can adjust the program as needed. For example, if you can only train 3 days a week, combine half of chest day and half of arm day, to form a

day chest-arm day.

There are many different training styles and variations you can do. Some examples include reverse pyramid, standard pyramid, straight sets, drop sets, rest pause training etc. However, studies have shown the greatest predictor of muscle growth is *volume*.

My sample training routine below will have a lot of volume, ensure you're working in recommended rep ranges, and contains a helpful progression model. With high volume and a good progression model, you will be packing on the muscle in no time.

Day 1: Chest
Barbell Bench Press:
- o   Set 1: 18-20 Reps
- o   Set 2: 13-15 Reps
- o   Set 3: 10-12 Reps
- o   Set 4: 6-8 Reps
- o   Set 5: 1-4 Reps
- o   Set 6: 1-4 Reps

Barbell Incline Press:
- o   Set 1: 18-20 Reps
- o   Set 2: 13-15 Reps
- o   Set 3: 10-12 Reps
- o   Set 4: 6-8 Reps
- o   Set 5: 1-4 Reps
- o   Set 6: 1-4 Reps

Incline Dumbbell Fly:
- o   Set 1: 18-20 Reps
- o   Set 2: 13-15 Reps
- o   Set 3: 10-12 Reps
- o   Set 4: 6-8 Reps
- o   Set 5: 1-4 Reps
- o   Set 6: 1-4 Reps

Cable Crossover:
- o   Set 1: 18-20 Reps
- o   Set 2: 13-15 Reps
- o   Set 3: 10-12 Reps
- o   Set 4: 6-8 Reps

- o Set 5: 1-4 Reps
- o Set 6: 1-4 Reps

Day 2: Arms

Close Grip Flat Bench:
- o Set 1: 18-20 Reps
- o Set 2: 13-15 Reps
- o Set 3: 10-12 Reps
- o Set 4: 8-10 Reps
- o Set 5: 6-8 Reps
- o Set 6: 6-8 Reps

Hammer Curls:
- o Set 1: 18-20 Reps
- o Set 2: 13-15 Reps
- o Set 3: 10-12 Reps
- o Set 4: 8-10 Reps
- o Set 5: 6-8 Reps
- o Set 6: 6-8 Reps

Triceps Pushdowns:
- o Set 1: 18-20 Reps
- o Set 2: 13-15 Reps
- o Set 3: 10-12 Reps
- o Set 4: 8-10 Reps
- o Set 5: 6-8 Reps
- o Set 6: 6-8 Reps

Preacher Curls:
- o Set 1: 18-20 Reps
- o Set 2: 13-15 Reps
- o Set 3: 10-12 Reps
- o Set 4: 8-10 Reps
- o Set 5: 6-8 Reps
- o Set 6: 6-8 Reps

Day 3: Legs

Body Weight Lunges (Warm Up):
- o Set 1: 10 steps
- o Set 2: 10 steps
- o Set 3: 10 steps

Barbell Squat:
- o   Set 1: 18-20 Reps
- o   Set 2: 13-15 Reps
- o   Set 3: 10-12 Reps
- o   Set 4: 8-10 Reps
- o   Set 5: 4-6 Reps
- o   Set 6: 4-6 Reps

Stiff Leg Deadlift:
- o   Set 1: 18-20 Reps
- o   Set 2: 13-15 Reps
- o   Set 3: 10-12 Reps
- o   Set 4: 8-10 Reps
- o   Set 5: 4-6 Reps
- o   Set 6: 4-6 Reps

Leg Press:
- o   Set 1: 18-20 Reps
- o   Set 2: 13-15 Reps
- o   Set 3: 10-12 Reps
- o   Set 4: 8-10 Reps
- o   Set 5: 4-6 Reps
- o   Set 6: 4-6 Reps

Walking Lunges:
- o   Set 1: 10 Steps
- o   Set 2: 15 Steps
- o   Set 3: 20 Steps
- o   Set 4: 25 Steps
- o   Set 5: 30 Steps
- o   Set 6: 40 Steps

Calf Press:
- o   Set 1: 18-20 Reps
- o   Set 2: 18-20 Reps
- o   Set 3: 13-15 Reps
- o   Set 4: 13-15 Reps
- o   Set 5: 10-12 Reps
- o   Set 6: 8-10 Reps

Day 4: Shoulders

Dumbbell Press:
- o Set 1: 18-20 Reps
- o Set 2: 13-15 Reps
- o Set 3: 10-12 Reps
- o Set 4: 8-10 Reps
- o Set 5: 4-6 Reps
- o Set 6: 4-6 Reps

Lateral Raise:
- o Set 1: 18-20 Reps
- o Set 2: 13-15 Reps
- o Set 3: 10-12 Reps
- o Set 4: 8-10 Reps
- o Set 5: 6-8 Reps
- o Set 6: 6-8 Reps

Barbell Shrugs:
- o Set 1: 18-20 Reps
- o Set 2: 13-15 Reps
- o Set 3: 10-12 Reps
- o Set 4: 8-10 Reps
- o Set 5: 6-8 Reps
- o Set 6: 6-8 Reps

Front Raise:
- o Set 1: 18-20 Reps
- o Set 2: 13-15 Reps
- o Set 3: 10-12 Reps
- o Set 4: 8-10 Reps
- o Set 5: 6-8 Reps
- o Set 6: 6-8 Reps

Day 5: Back
Deadlift:
- o Set 1: 18-20 Reps
- o Set 2: 13-15 Reps
- o Set 3: 10-12 Reps
- o Set 4: 6-8 Reps
- o Set 5: 1-4 Reps
- o Set 6: 1-4 Reps

Lat Pulldown:

- o   Set 1: 18-20 Reps
- o   Set 2: 13-15 Reps
- o   Set 3: 10-12 Reps
- o   Set 4: 6-8 Reps
- o   Set 5: 1-4 Reps
- o   Set 6: 1-4 Reps

Seated Row:
- o   Set 1: 18-20 Reps
- o   Set 2: 13-15 Reps
- o   Set 3: 10-12 Reps
- o   Set 4: 6-8 Reps
- o   Set 5: 1-4 Reps
- o   Set 6: 1-4 Reps

Bent Over Row:
- o   Set 1: 18-20 Reps
- o   Set 2: 13-15 Reps
- o   Set 3: 10-12 Reps
- o   Set 4: 6-8 Reps
- o   Set 5: 1-4 Reps
- o   Set 6: 1-4 Reps

Weight lifting pro-tips:
1. Always ensure you are in control of the weight for the entire movement. Don't swing.
2. Keep a journal. Tracking your weights will help you remember your past week's lifts, which will help you know if you need to move up in weight or reps.
3. Choose weights that will ensure you reach failure at the given rep range.
4. Rest around 2m in between each set.
5. Progression Model: Push yourself to failure. If at any point you are able to push past the given amount of reps. Go up by 2.5-5lbs next week for that specific set.

Goals

The following section will help you choose the nutrition and workout plan that best fits you. There are four strategies to choose from. Just choose the one that relates most to your goals.

In this section, a beginner will be defined as someone who has been lifting for 1-6 months. Intermediate to advanced will be defined as someone who has been lifting for over 6 months.

Strategy #1 - For Beginners: I want to lose fat and build muscle.

I recommend that you choose the "extreme weight loss protocol" and the "weight lifting" approach. For faster fat loss results, add cardio.

Strategy #2 - For Intermediate - Advanced: I don't care about muscle; I just want to lose fat.

I recommend you choose the "extreme weight loss protocol" and the "cardio" approach.

Strategy #3 - For Intermediate - Advanced: I want to lose fat and maintain muscle.

Depending on how much fat you want to lose, I recommend you choose the "recomposition" or "extreme weight loss" protocol, paired with the "weight lifting" approach.

Strategy #4 - For Intermediate - Advanced: I want to build lean muscle.

I recommend you choose the "lean bulk" protocol, along with the "weight training" approach.

Note: I know some of you in the Intermediate - Advanced category would like to know what you must do to *lose fat and build muscle simultaneously*. I still believe this is almost impossible to do without taking performance-enhancing drugs. However, here are some suggestions if you fall into this category:

1. Focus on Strategy #3 and choose "extreme weight loss" for your nutrition protocol. This will help you lose weight and get to a low body fat level quickly.

Once you are down to about 6-10% body fat, switch to Strategy #4. This is what I did to lose weight and it worked wonders. Once you are down to 6-10% body fat, your progress is no longer hiding behind a layer of fat, making your results much more visible and enjoyable.

CHAPTER 9: TIPS, TRICKS, MYTHS, & QUESTIONS

Tips
1: Drink coffee.

- One technique to keeping your appetite under control is drinking coffee when you wake up, and then again when you get hungry. Not only will this give you insane focus, but it will suppress your appetite, making the fast much easier. Coffee has no calories, which means it's free to drink during your fast.

2: Eat an apple.

- It can be hard to stick to a diet when you are eating a lower calorie protocol like the "extreme weight loss" protocol I mentioned earlier. If this is the case, eat an apple when you first get hungry. An apple is only 100 calories and will restore your glycogen stores to ensure that you can push your first meal another 2 hours. I typically have an apple around 2pm after my two cups of coffee.

3: Expect some confused looks from others.

- Your friends and family might not get this whole intermittent fasting thing at first. I have met people for breakfast countless times while only ordering coffee but no food. When their food comes, they look at me as if I'm crazy. But that's okay! When someone asks, explain what you're doing. Otherwise I don't worry about it. Simply embrace the questions, then embrace the results.

4: Keep yourself busy.

- Sometimes it's hard to tell the difference between hunger and boredom. If you are struggling initially, keep yourself busy. Go for a walk. Do some work. I have actually found that I have the best concentration while fasting.

5: Drink water or green tea.

- When fasting, you can still drink as many zero-calorie beverages as you want. Staying hydrated will also make your fast easier.

6: Keep track of your strength.

- If you are fearful of losing muscle while dieting, simply track your strength when training. If your strength and volume stay the same and you are eating adequate protein (1g per pound of bodyweight), then you most likely aren't losing any muscle.

7: Track your calories and measurements.

- Knowing how many calories to eat can often be a bit of a guessing game. This tip will help your gain clarity.
- Once you've set your calories, stick to them to the best of your ability. Once a week make sure you weigh yourself first thing in the morning and take your body measurements.
  o If your waist has stayed the same but your weight has gone up, you have picked up muscle.
  o If your waist stays the same and your weight has gone down, you have most likely lost muscle. In this case, up your calories by 100.
  o If your waist goes down and your weight has gone down, you have lost fat.
  o Keep testing every week until you are at an optimal level.

8: Don't lose your head.

- Keep it simple. Intermittent fasting does not need to be a complicated thing. If you break your fast half an hour early, or miss your eating window by an hour or two, that's ok. Life is crazy. But your diet doesn't have to be. Just do your best to listen to your body and go with the flow.

Motivation
1: Track your measurements.

- As I said before, this will ensure you are able to see your progress.

2: Use the mirror, not the scale.

- The scale tends to freak people out. If your progress looks good in the mirror (or in your progress pictures), what the scale says doesn't really matter.

3: Start with a friend.
- Finding an accountability partner will greatly increase your chance of success.

4: Use a variety of foods.
- It's ok to still enjoy food. And it's okay to change things up. As long as you consistently hit your macro targets, everything will work out.

Myths
1: You need to eat breakfast to start your metabolism.
- Studies have shown that there is no need to "start" your metabolism. When you don't have food in your stomach, your body will continue getting its fuel from the fat you've stored.

2: It is possible to damage your metabolism.
- It's simply not true. I spoke about this at length in **chapter 6**. I would encourage you refer to the **common questions** section there.

3: You have to eat 6 meals a day to burn fat.
- When you eat a meal, your body needs to burn extra calories to process that meal. Therefore, a lot of books will tell you to eat all the time so your metabolism can be firing all day long. This is false.
- Studies have shown that whether you eat 2,500 calories spread through the day, or 2,500 calories in a small window, your body will burn the same amount of calories processing the food.

Drawbacks
I haven't found many negative side effects when it comes to intermittent fasting. The biggest concern people have is that fasting will lead to lower energy, focus, and feeling hungry all the time.

However, I have found that while some adjustment may be required initially, most people are able to make the change fairly easily and effectively.

You can retrain your body not to expect food every three hours. Think about our ancestors who had to hunt for their food. Their bodies were quite used to not eating every 3 hours. Over time, our bodies can adapt in the same way too.

Note: If you have issues with diabetes, hypoglycemia, or have issues with blood sugar regulation, please consult a medical professional before attempting to start intermittent fasting.

Common Questions
1: Does intermittent fasting effect men and women differently?
- Yes, intermittent fasting can affect men and woman differently. One study showed that intermittent fasting improved insulin sensitivity in males, however females didn't see the same results. But IF is safe to try for both men and women. The best thing you can do is give it a try, monitor your results, and decide from there.

2: Will I get hungry?
- Initially you may. If you eat often, you have trained your body to be fed often. But if you can train your body to be fed often, then you can train your body to fast as well.

3: Why was I told to consume 30g of protein every few hours?
- This is a lie that supplement companies have sold us for years to influence product sales. Maybe you've heard your body can only digest 30g of protein at a time, and if you don't continually have protein you will lose muscle. This simply isn't true. But these companies know eating 30g of protein every few hours is difficult so most people will buy their supplements to help.
- In this study, we see that our bodies are able to preserve muscle while fasting, which means you don't need protein every few hours to preserve muscle. Additionally, protein absorption can take place over many hours after protein is consumed.

4: I've been doing intermittent fasting, but I'm still not losing weight. What do I do?
- **Count and cut your calories**: If you have been following intermittent fasting but are not losing weight, I would encourage you to start counting calories closely. Count *everything* that goes into your mouth, even that handful of nuts or couple bites of a snack. Most of the time people are blowing their diets on the little things they are eating every day and not counting.

  Remember, intermittent fasting is a dieting pattern, not a diet in itself. That being said, calories still matter. If you eat more calories than you burn, you will pick up weight. But the inverse of that is also true.

- **2: Reverse diet:** If your calorie intake is already very low (1,200 calories for women, 1,500 for men), I would also recommend that you refer to **"Reverse Dieting"** in chapter 6 for a more in-depth look at this question.

- **3: Consult a doctor.** If you have carefully counted your calories, followed the "reverse dieting" protocol successfully, and re-entered a fat loss phase and still aren't looking weight, I would encourage you to see a doctor. There could be a medical issue that needs to be addressed. One of the most common yet often misdiagnosed conditions is hypothyroidism. Most of the time the problem is not counting calories, but if you feel like this might be you, I would encourage you to research hypothyroidism online and consult your doctor.

5: What if my body goes into "starvation mode" when I start fasting?

People falsely believe that if they don't eat for 16-24 hours, their bodies will enter "starvation mode," slowing down their metabolism and storing fat as soon as food is consumed. But studies show us that the earliest signs of a lowered metabolic rate from fasting happen after at least 60 hours without food. Some studies showed that metabolic rate wasn't actually impacted until 72-96 hours had passed. Bottom line: intermittent fasting doesn't require you to fast for 72 hours, or even 60 hours. If you are following any of the fasting methods I mentioned in **Chapter 4**, your body won't enter into starvation mode.

CHAPTER 10: YOUR ACTION PLAN

Where to Start

We have covered a lot of information in this book that I hope has been helpful. My goal is to cut through all the noise when it comes to health and fitness. There are all sorts of theories and hypotheticals for fitness that are available. But I want to help you achieve your goals in the most efficient and effective way.

More than ever, I'm also convinced that if you follow this plan, there is no limit to what you can achieve.

How to Incorporate Fasting into a Daily Schedule

Step 1: Make a decision to pursue a healthy lifestyle. Tell your friends so they can help by holding you accountable. Decide that this is a MUST for you. Think in the long-term and set some process-orientated goals. **(Chapter 1)**

Step 2: Pick an intermittent fasting method. Choose one that will work best with your current lifestyle. **(Chapter 4)**

Step 3: Based on your goals, choose the best nutrition protocol for you. **(Chapter 6)**

Step 4: Choose an exercise plan that will best fit your lifestyle and help you achieve the body you desire. **(Chapter 8)**

Step 5: Start following the plan, adjusting as you go along. Track your weight and measurements. Aim for small weekly wins that will lead to long-term success.

Step 6: Email me if you have any questions - noahlively.ebooks@publishingwhale.com. Fitness coaching is infamously expensive. But because you made the decision to invest in yourself when you bought this book, I want to invest in you for FREE! All I ask is if this book has been helpful to you, would you be so kind as to leave a review on Amazon? Chances are, if this book has helped you, it can help someone else.

Take a moment and do that right now.

Here is a link right to the review page: http://amzn.to/2lt7v5c

CONCLUSION

I want to thank you and congratulate you for getting this far. Did you know that only 10% of people who buy books get past the first chapter?

If you made it this far, it shows that you are committed to making a change and pursuing your goals. I couldn't be more proud of you.

My goal has always been to add value and improve your life. In this book, I set out to teach you about intermittent fasting but I hoped to do a bit more than that. I want you to understand fat loss and muscle building. I want to give you motivation and confidence that *you can do this*.

I want to give you tools and protocols to help you. Male or female. Losing weight or building muscle. YOU.

If this has been helpful to you, would you consider taking a moment and leaving a review on Amazon? There are a lot of books available about intermittent fasting but unfortunately, many of them are feeding people false information.

When you leave an honest review, it ensures this book can get into as many hands as possible and more people can achieve the same results you are about to see.

Your review will help others who are frustrated with their health. Maybe others just like you, who have tried everything but haven't seen any progress.

Go to this link to leave a review: http://amzn.to/2lt7v5c

If you find anything in this book to be false or disagreeable, please email me at noahlively.ebooks@publishingwhale.com. Accuracy is very important to me so I will do everything I can to correct any mistakes or further help you understand this process.

Wishing you ever-increasing success as you achieve your dreams,

Noah

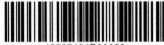